SUGAR DETOX FOR BEGINNERS

A Quick Start Guide to Bust Sugar Cravings, Stop Sugar Addiction, Increase Energy, and Lose Weight with the Sugar Detox Diet

Including a 7-Day Meal Plan and Delicious Sugar Free "Detox Friendly" Recipes

Gina Crawford

D1304471

Copyright © 2014 by Gina Crawford

Evita Publishing, PO Box 306, Station A, Vancouver Island, BC V9W 5B1 Canada

IMPORTANT

The information in this book reflects the author's research, experiences and opinions and is not intended to replace medical advice.

Before beginning this or any nutritional or exercise regimen, consult your physician to be sure it is appropriate for you. Ask for a physical stress test.

Table of Contents

Introduction

Thank you for purchasing *Sugar Detox for Beginners: A Quick Start Guide to Bust Sugar Cravings, Increase Energy and Lose Weight with the Sugar Detox Diet.* Also, congratulations for taking the first step to taming your sugar cravings and improving your health.

Learning how to get healthier doesn't have to take a ton of time. I know you're busy yet you want to know the best, most effective way to detox your body from the harmful effects of sugar.

This book has been designed with you in mind. It is a no-fluff, to-the-point quick read that is jam-packed with the necessary information you need to curb your sugar cravings FAST by applying the sugar detox diet to your life.

In this book you will learn everything you need to know about applying a 21-day, 7-day or a 3-day sugar detox to your life. Choose whichever one suits your lifestyle best.

You will also learn the effects of bad sugars on the body, how the sugar detox can help you lose weight, why sugar causes disease, good foods to eat while on a sugar detox, foods to avoid, the symptoms and benefits of a sugar detox, the difference between a natural sweetener, a naturally derived sweetener and an artificial sweetener, how to dine out during your detox, how to reintroduce sugar, how to maintain a limited sugar lifestyle and more!

As an added bonus, this book also includes Sugar Free "Detox Friendly" breakfast, lunch, dinner, salad, soup, side dish, dessert and snack recipes as well as a 7-day sample meal plan.

The goal of this book is to enable you to dive right into a sugar detox that will eradicate your sugar cravings, increase your energy, help you lose weight and transform your health!

Congratulations again for taking the initiative to control your sweet tooth rather than allowing it to dominate you. Your body will thank you for applying this detox to your life! Hope you enjoy the book and get a lot out of it!

Chapter 1

Your Body and Sugar

What is sugar?

Sugar is the general name for short chain soluble carbohydrates found in food. These sweet tasting carbohydrates are made of carbon, hydrogen, and oxygen.

How is sugar made?

Sugar farmers grow and harvest sugar cane and sugar beet plants. In the harvesting process farmers extract the sugar juice from each plant then refine it by running it through a series of wash and dry cycles that turn the juice into fine sugar crystals.

These sugar crystals are sold as unbleached, not heavily refined higher molasses content crystals commonly known as raw sugar. Or the sugar crystals are sold as bleached, further refined lower molasses content crystals commonly known as table sugar.

What is sugar used for in the human body?

Glucose, a simple sugar, is the body's key source of energy. It is also the primary source of energy for the brain. If glucose is lacking, psychological processes that require mental effort are impaired. The central nervous system runs on glucose throughout the day and our muscles require glucose in order to function at their best during strenuous workouts.

Red blood cells use glucose for energy. During pregnancy, glucose can help form cells and produce milk.

To conserve fuel the body stores extra glucose that is not required for energy as a compound called glycogen. Through a process called glycogenesis the liver makes glycogen chains up to thousands of glucose molecules long.

The body then breaks down glycogen into units of glucose that it can use for energy when primary sources are not available. This occurs during sleep, meals, and throughout workouts to prevent dangerous drops in blood sugar.

The human body can't function without sugar. Why is it then that sugar receives such harsh criticism? It's not because of the good that sugar does, rather it's because of the lack of nutritional value that simple sugar contains.

The difference between simple and complex carbohydrates

All carbohydrates are composed of units of sugar. Carbohydrates exist in all foods except fats (like oils) and animal protein. What makes various carbohydrates different from each other is the amount of sugar units that they contain.

Carbohydrates can be divided into three subcategories:

1. Simple carbohydrates (otherwise known as simple sugars)

2. Complex carbohydrates (commonly known as starches)

3. Dietary fiber

Bad carbohydrates

Bad carbohydrates are simple carbohydrates that are made up of only one or two units of sugar. Their *simple* structure enables the body to break them down and digest them too quickly to offer the proper nutrients and energy to the body that it needs. The rapid digestion of simple carbohydrates causes them to be released into the blood stream quickly therefore causing a spike in the body's energy level followed by a crash in energy.

White bread, white rice, alcohol, soft drinks, cakes, cookies and chips are examples of bad carbohydrates that are full of empty calories.

Lactose, fructose and sucrose are also simple sugars. These should be avoided as they offer no nutritional value.

Good carbohydrates

Good carbohydrates are complex carbohydrates that contain more than two units of sugar linked together. Complex carbohydrates can have three to millions of units of sugar linked together. Their complexity causes the body to take longer to digest them therefore releasing glucose into the blood stream more slowly and evenly than simple carbohydrates.

Dietary fiber is another kind of complex carbohydrate. Though it does not act as a source of energy for the body it provides many other positive benefits.

Fiber is classified by nutritionists as either insoluble fiber or soluble fiber. This is based on whether it dissolves in water. Both insoluble and soluble fibers are incapable of being broken down by the body's digestive enzymes. For this reason, fiber adds no additional calories to your diet and it cannot be converted to glucose.

Fiber is valuable to the human body because you can't digest it. Insoluble fiber is a natural laxative. It can be found in whole wheat, whole grains, bran, beans, carrots, beets, cabbage, plant stems and leaves. It absorbs water, helps you feel full longer and it helps move solid materials through your intestines quickly, preventing digestive disorders such as constipation and diverticulitis.

Soluble fiber found in fruits, barley, beans, oats, rice, seeds and seaweed helps to lower the amount of cholesterol circulating in the blood.

This makes soluble fiber a natural aid in preventing heart disease.

Not all simple sugars are bad

All *bad sugars* are *simple*, but here's where it gets tricky. Not all *simple sugars* are considered *bad* because it depends where the sugar comes from. For example, beans, nuts, whole grains, fruits, and vegetables all contain simple sugars but these sugars are part of what is considered 'whole foods'. This means that they don't just contain sugar they also contain minerals, proteins, and vitamins. This makes them more than just empty calories.

All of these sugars are 'good sugars' and they occur naturally in the foods that most of us eat every day. This is why they are commonly called *natural sugars*.

It's the teaspoon of refined table sugar added to your coffee or the little bit added to your cooking that is considered *bad*. This "added sugar" as the health industry calls it, contains no minerals or fiber, just empty calories.

The effects of bad sugars on the body

Sugar consumption is at an all time high and it is affecting our health in a negative way. In fact, statistics say that the average American consumes more than 156 pounds of added sugar every year. The largest source of Americans sugar calorie intake comes from high fructose corn syrup.

Soft drinks, sports drinks, and fruit juices are all loaded with sugar. There are also many foods that contain hidden sugars. Processed foods like pretzels, bottled pasta sauce, bologna, Worcestershire sauce, barbeque sauce and cheese spread also contain a lot of sugar.

Nowadays most infant formula contains the sugar equivalent of one can of Coke. Babies therefore are being metabolically programmed to be sugar addicts from day one.

Most people associate high sugar intake with weight gain. They don't realize however that weight gain is only one negative side effect of sugar.

Sugar can be extremely damaging to the body because it can cause all kinds of life threatening diseases. It can also have damaging outer and inner physical effects that are not life threatening but that do inhibit the quality of one's life.

Why sugar causes disease

An excessive intake of sugar causes extra sugar molecules to remain in the bloodstream. Sugars that are left unused in the bloodstream have to go somewhere so they latch on to protein molecules throughout the entire body.

These protein-sugar complexes called *advanced glycation end products* cause massive inflammation in the body as well as tissue damage and premature aging. Many of the diseases that we associate with aging are actually caused by this process.

Normally, inflammation is a natural immune response. Pain, swelling, and redness are usually all positive signs that the body is working to repair tissue and heal a wound. This is called acute inflammation.

Chronic inflammation is when your body is no longer capable of turning off the inflammatory response and it begins attacking healthy tissue mistaking it for something harmful.

In 2004, Time Magazine called inflammation "The Secret Killer" because once it silently starts running out of control it can damage the intestinal lining and cause digestive problems, it can damage arteries in the heart and cause heart disease, and it can damage joints and cause rheumatoid arthritis.

Obviously, things like sleep deprivation, stress, bacteria, viruses, and environmental poisons (to name a few) also contribute to chronic inflammation. Controlling sugar intake is just one of the ways that you can consciously avoid the risk of developing diseases due to chronic inflammation.

A high sugar diet can provoke the following undesirable conditions and maladies.

Weight Gain

Today, 32% of Americans suffer from obesity and another one third is considered over-weight. This number has more than doubled since 1975 when the obesity rate in America was only 15 %. Carrying excess weight increases your risk of heart disease, diabetes and kidney disease.

Consuming sugar that is not in the 'whole foods' category means consuming empty calories. Empty calories means....you guessed it, weight gain!

When you eat too much sugar the pancreas releases insulin to handle the rush of sugars entering the body. This is like an alarm to the liver alerting it to turn the complex and simple sugars into glucose for our bodies to use as energy.

If not all of the glucose produced is used the liver works again to change the glucose into glycogen. It then sends it out to be stored in the muscles and fat tissue.

Glycogen is eventually used for energy. That's a good thing right? There's just one problem. The body only stores 12 hours worth of glycogen and the rest is converted by the liver to nothing but fat.

The problem with fructose

Sugar and high fructose corn syrup contain both glucose and fructose. Fructose is not a natural part of our metabolism and few cells in the body can use it. It is metabolized by the liver and there it gets turned into fat which is then secreted into the blood.

Fructose causes insulin resistance and raises insulin levels in the blood which selectively deposit energy from foods into fat cells. This causes weight gain.

Fructose also causes the brain to resist leptin which means that the brain can't see all the stored fat in the body. This makes it think that the body is starving. As a result, an urge is triggered to keep eating when you don't need to eat. This results in weight gain.

Fructose also doesn't make you feel full after meals. It only leads to an increase in calorie intake and ultimately weight gain.

Skin problems

Dermatologist Dr. Patricia Ferris, a specialist in aging skin noticed that many women seeking a cure for their aging skin had one thing in common. Their skin did not have the usual symptoms of sun-damage that she suspected, yet it was very wrinkled and had a significant loss of elasticity.

The one common thread with all of these women was that they had a diet that consisted of poor nutrition and excessive sugar consumption.

"Research shows that a diet laced with sugar and refined carbohydrates can age the skin more than a lifetime of lying in the sun" said Dr. Ferris.

The process that links sugar and premature aging is called glycation. As mentioned above, glycation occurs when blood sugar levels are excessively high. Sugar molecules bond with other components in the blood and form protein-sugar complexes known as advanced glycation end-products, or AGE's. This triggers an inflammatory response causing tissue damage and premature aging.

The molecules in your face that promote a youthful glow are very sensitive to sugar. When collagen and elastin molecules are turned into AGE's their soft and supple fibers become rigid. This causes saggy, baggy, wrinkled skin.

When you eat sugar and refined carbs you deliberately attack your own collagen and elastin therefore destroying your own appearance of youth. This also causes defects in your complexion like dryness, vulnerability to infection and acne.

Dr. Ferris recommends that one of the best things you can do for your skin is replace sugar with apples and other foods containing antiglycating antioxidants which are chemicals that fight the glycation process naturally.

Diabetes

The Center for Disease Control has estimated that by the year 2050 one in three Americans will have diabetes. This can be prevented if we eat better, exercise more and lower our consumption of sugar.

Diabetes, or diabetes mellitus, is a common disease caused by a high sugar and high fat diet. Diabetes occurs when the pancreas fails to produce adequate insulin when the blood sugar rises.

A concentrated amount of sugar sent into the system causes the body to go into shock from the rapid rise in the blood sugar level. Eventually the pancreas wears out from overwork and diabetes sets in.

Being overweight and eating foods high in simple sugars are both factors that contribute to this disease.

Badly controlled diabetes can lead to mental health disorders, hearing loss, stroke, eye complications, and general circulation issues to the extremities of the body.

Hypoglycemia

Hypoglycemia occurs when the pancreas overreacts to a large amount of sugar in the blood and releases an excess of insulin. This leaves an individual feeling tired because the blood sugar level sinks lower than it should.

Heart Disease

Studies show that diets high in sugar increase the body's risk of developing heart disease especially in women. While the exact amount of sugar needed to cause this change hasn't been determined by professionals, something as simple as one soft drink a day has been proven to double or even triple the risk for some people.

With sugar contributing to high blood pressure and unhealthy cholesterol levels, it's only logical that heart disease would be close behind as a result of a high sugar diet.

Lack of focus

Another serious problem with sugar is the various levels of mental issues that it can cause. The human brain is very sensitive and reacts to quick chemical changes within the body.

One of the keys to efficient brain function is glutamic acid which is a compound commonly found in many vegetables. When sugar is consumed, the bacteria in the intestines which manufacture vitamin B complexes begin to die. When the B vitamin complex levels decline, the glutamic acid is not processed and this results in sleepiness, as well as a decreased ability for short-term memory function and numerical calculative abilities.

It also leads to a confused mental state and has also been associated with juvenile criminal behavior. In fact, Dr. Alexander Schauss in his *Diet, Crime and Delinquency* book says that "many mental ward and prison inmates are sugarholics and experience erratic emotional outbreaks following a sugar binge."

Research also shows that sugar can cause 'free radicals' in the brain that make it difficult to focus on both menial and complicated tasks. It can also make it difficult to listen and pay attention properly.

Insomnia

With sugars causing insulin to be produced by the pancreas and simple sugars causing bursts of insulin to be produced by the pancreas, it can be hard for our bodies to adjust to these significant highs and lows.

One of the functions of the stress hormone cortisol is to regulate the body's glucose levels to ensure that the body's muscles, heart, and vital organs have enough glucose (energy) to continue doing what they do best... keeping you alive.

Highs and lows of insulin and glucose can increase cortisol in the body making the body physically stressed out, complete with sweaty palms and a pounding heart. This makes it difficult to sleep because your body feels like it's running a marathon.

Dental problems

Sugar makes the blood very thick and sticky. This inhibits the blood flow into the tiny capillaries that supply the gums and teeth with vital nutrients. This causes gum disease as well as teeth that are deficient of necessary nutrients.

Chewing gum can also be harmful not only because of the sugar content in gum that damages teeth but because the teeth and jaws were never designed to put up with more than a few minutes of solid gum chewing per day. People who enjoy chewing gum often chew for an average of two hours daily. This amount of gum chewing results in excessive wear and tear on the jawbone, gum tissue and lower molars. It can also change the alignment of the jaw.

Other sugar disorders

Sugar also plays a major role in atherosclerosis, Alzheimer's cataracts, depression and other diseases.

Chapter 2

Sugar and Addiction

Sugar Addiction

Many nutrition experts say that refined sugar is as harmful as a drug particularly when it is consumed in the quantities that the average American consumes it. In the refining process white sugar is stripped down to nothing but the carbohydrates pure calories. It contains no fats, enzymes, vitamins, minerals or proteins. This makes it a non-food. It is simply a pure chemical derived from plant sources that many say is purer than cocaine.

Studies show that sugar actually causes the brain to react in a similar way that it does to opiates like heroin or morphine. Sugar can create a euphoric effect on the mind and body. We naturally try to achieve that same 'euphoric' feeling every time we consume sugar, and like all drugs it forces us to consume more sugar to create the same 'high' we had previously on a smaller amount of sugar.

Experiments done on both animals and humans alike show that the sudden removal of sugar in the body results in withdrawal symptoms that are similar to someone getting off of a narcotic. The chemical dependency of the body on sugar suffers when it is removed and results in anxiety, cravings and even 'the shakes' in the addict.

A healthy properly functioning digestive system can digest and eliminate two to four teaspoons of sugar daily without any problems. One 12 ounce can of Coke contains 10.5 teaspoons of sugar. That doesn't even include other (sugary) foods or drinks that would be consumed in a day along with that one can of Coke. Truth is the average person consumes twenty six teaspoons of sugar a day. That's six to twelve times more than the body can handle.

The National Health Service recommends:

70 grams of sugar a day for men

50 grams of sugar a day for women

Are you addicted to sugar?

Could you be addicted to sugar and not know it? Some researchers say that most of us are and it's not that hard to tell. Ask yourself these questions to see if you might be addicted to sugar.

When thinking about cutting sugar out of your diet, do you worry about cutting out some specific foods that you eat regularly?

Do you eat certain foods even if you aren't hungry and mostly because you crave them?

Do you overeat often? Do you feel tired or maybe even sluggish after you overeat?

Do you have a hard time stopping at just one scoop of ice cream?

Do you have health problems as a result of your diet but can't seem to make the changes you need to help yourself?

Do you find it hard to walk past a sugary treat without indulging in one?

Have you unconsciously set up routines around sugar like having a donut with your morning coffee?

Are there times in your day when you feel that you can't make it through without a blast of sugar?

Do you develop mood swings and headaches if you have to go for a day without sugar?

Chapter 3

Sugar Detox

Kicking the Habit

What is a detox?

Detox, short for detoxification, is a natural way of cleansing the body of harmful toxins that enter the body through environmental pollutants or diet. If left in the body, they can cause adverse effects, disease and death.

During a detox, the lungs, skin, kidneys, intestines, liver and lymphatic system work together to turn toxins into less harmful compounds that can be eliminated from the body.

A detox diet is a way of removing environmental and dietary toxins from the body. There are three goals of a detox diet:

To increase the intake of vitamins, minerals, antioxidants and nutrients that can help the body repair and cleanse itself

To minimize the amount of chemicals going into the body by eating organic foods

28

To increase the intake of high fiber foods and water that enable the body to excrete harmful toxins

Why the Sugar Detox Diet?

Doctors all over the country are claiming that the only way to kick the curse of sugar on your body is to allow your body to undergo a natural process of eliminating the toxin (sugar) from your body. It's like ripping the band-aid off.

A detox is the quickest way to effectively remove sugar from your system, break the dangerous cycle of unhealthy sugar cravings and give you a fresh start to establish dietary order.

Remember, before you do anything, run your plan by your physician. So long as you aren't pregnant, nursing, or have major issues with insulin or blood sugar, a sugar detox should work for you.

How will the Sugar Detox Diet help you lose weight?

Remember that problem of glucose being converted into glycogen and then being stored in the body? When no sugars are available for your body to burn as energy, the liver takes on the task of creating sugar by itself! How? By taking the converted glycogen stored in your body fat and changing it back to glucose. This breaks down the fat and turns it into burnable sugar for energy!

Chapter 4

The 21 Day Sugar Detox Diet

How does the Sugar Detox Diet work?

Follow these four steps diligently to get the best results from the diet:

*Remove all sugar and simple carbs from your diet for **21 days in a row**.*

Don't eat anything on the 'Foods to avoid' list.

Only eat foods on the 'Good Foods' list.

If you mess up and give in, start over from day one.

On the next few pages you will find a list of foods to eat and foods to avoid on the sugar detox diet. Make sure to eat lots of the good foods for 21 days and stay away from the bad foods. Being diligent about eating the right foods is the key to detoxifying your body. Also, remember to keep yourself well hydrated through the sugar detox.

GOOD FOODS

ANIMAL PROTEINS LIKE:

Beef

Bison

Chicken

Deli and cured meats like prosciutto, pancetta, bacon etc.

Eggs

Lamb

Pork

Sausages

Shellfish (shrimp, mussels, clams, oysters) and other seafood

Tuna

Turkey

Veal

White fish

Wild salmon

VEGETABLES THAT ARE NOT STARCHY:

Alfalfa sprouts

All leafy greens

Artichokes

Asparagus

Avocado

Bamboo shoots

Bean Sprouts

Bok Choy

Broccoli

Brussels sprouts

Cabbage

Carrots

Cauliflower

Celery

Chard

Chinese cabbage

Collards

Cucumber

Daikon

Eggplant

Fennel

Garlic

Ginger

Green beans

Jicama

Kale

Leeks

Lettuce

Mushrooms

Okra

Onions

Parsnips

Peppers (all kinds)

Radicchio

Radishes

Rhubarb

Rutabaga

Shallots/green onions

Snap peas

Snow peas

Spaghetti squash

Spinach

Swiss chard

Tomato

Turnips

Yellow squash

Water chestnuts

Watercress

Zucchini

FRUITS:

Lemons

Limes

NUTS:

Nuts and seeds: whole, ground into flour, or processed into butters

Brazil nuts, walnuts, hazelnuts, almond flour, almond meal, pecans, macadamias, pine nuts, and pistachios (no peanuts or cashews)

Coconut in all of its unsweetened forms: coconut, coconut flour, dried coconut. Coconut sugar is not allowed

SEEDS:

Apricot seeds

Chia seeds

Cocoa (100%) is acceptable.

Flax seeds

Hemp seeds

Pumpkin seeds

Sesame seeds

Sunflower seeds

Tahini

FATS:

Saturated fats from animal sources - butter,
ghee, duck fat, chicken fat, lamb fat, lard.
Grass-fed and organic are best.

Saturated fats from plant sources - coconut oil,
palm oil. Organic and unrefined are best.

COOKING OILS:

Bacon or pork fat

Beef fat

Butter/ghee (clarified butter)

Cocoa butter

Coconut oil

Duck fat

Palm oil

OILS FOR COLD USE ONLY:

Avocado oil

Extra virgin olive oil

Flaxseed oil – consume in very limited amounts due to polyunsaturated fatty acids

Nut oils - macadamia oil, walnut oil, pecan oil

Rice bran oil

BEVERAGES:

Coffee, teas (green, black, herbal, white) – without sugar

Nut milks – unsweetened almond milk, coconut milk

Water, club soda, seltzer, mineral water

CONDIMENTS, MISCELLANEOUS:

All herbs are allowed – For pre-mixed blends check for hidden ingredients

All spices are allowed – For pre-mixed blends check for hidden ingredients

Capers, fish sauce, hot sauce, tomato paste, gluten-free mustard, baking soda, coconut aminos, kelp flakes, Japanese edible seaweed

Homemade broth, ketchup, mayonnaise, salad dressings

Hummus – make sure it is made using cauliflower

Vanilla extract, vanilla bean extract, almond extract

Vinegars – Balsamic, apple cider, red wine, white, sherry and distilled

FOODS TO AVOID:

Use the "When in doubt leave it out" policy when it comes to knowing what foods to avoid. If a food tastes sweet and it's not on the good foods list, leave it out.

REFINED CARBOHYDRATES:

Breads of any kind

Cereal, granola

Chips

Crackers

Pastas (including couscous and orzo)

Processed grains – rice cakes, oats, popcorn

Sweet treats like cupcakes, brownies, candy, cake, cookies, pastries, muffins

PROCESSED FOODS:

Cut out all processed and genetically modified foods

STARCHY VEGETABLES:

Corn

Grits

Polenta

Yams

Plantain

Sweet potatoes and regular potatoes

Tapioca

GRAINS:

Anything made from wheat, barley, kamut,
spelt, rye

Flours made from grains or beans (wheat flour,
lentil flour, chickpea flour, spelt flour)

LEGUMES:

Beans and soy products

NUTS:

Cashews

Peanuts

FATS AND OILS:

Buttery spreads like "I Can't Believe it's not Butter" or Benecol

Highly processed unsaturated oils like corn oil, canola oil, sunflower oil, vegetable oil, grape seed oil, soybean oil, rice bran oil and safflower oil that oxidize easily in air, heat or light

Hydrogenated or partly hydrogenated oils

Margarine

SUGARS OR SWEETENERS:

No sugars are allowed

No natural sweeteners, naturally derived sweeteners or artificial sweeteners of any kind are allowed

No coconut sugar

Products that say "sugar free," "diet" or "artificially sweetened"

DRINKS:

Alcohol

Juice and other sweet tasting drinks (excluding herbal teas)

Milk and dairy products

Protein powders that have more than one
ingredient

Sodas (including diet sodas)

CONDIMENTS, MISCELLANEOUS:

Hummus made from chickpeas or beans

Soy sauce

Store bought broth, ketchup, mayonnaise,
salad dressings

Chapter 5

The 3 Day Sugar Detox

If you want a sugar detox that is shorter than 21 days then commit to this simple three day sugar detox that follows the most basic rules:

No fruit (aside from limes and lemons)

No starches

No wheat

No dairy

No added sugars

Nutritionist Brooke Alpert and dermatologist Dr. Patricia Farris developed this simple 'cold turkey' way to cut your sugar strings.

Alpert and Farris say that you can begin to reverse the signs of premature aging and weight gain caused by sugar in just three days with this fast track sugar detox. They also claim that this mini-detox can help you break free of sugar addiction immediately.

After the three day sugar detox Alpert and Farris recommend following a four-week eating plan with sugar free recipes.

For a good batch of sugar free recipes I would recommend my book *Sugar Free Recipes: Speedy and Easy 30 MINUTE Sugar Free Recipes for Breakfast, Lunch, Dinner and Dessert* available on Amazon.

3 Day Sugar Detox

DAY ONE

Breakfast - Three scrambled eggs

Mid-morning snack - A handful of nuts (no peanuts or cashews)

Lunch - Poached chicken breast with mixed greens and half an avocado

Afternoon snack - Sliced peppers with two tablespoons of spinach hummus

Dinner - Edamame along with salmon and stir-fried broccoli and mushrooms

DAY TWO

Breakfast - Sautéed spinach with three scrambled eggs

Snack - A handful of nuts (no peanuts or cashews)

Lunch - Tuna Niçoise salad (see recipe in Chapter 14 under Salads)

Snack - Sliced peppers with hummus (not made from chickpeas or beans)

Dinner - Pork tenderloin sautéed Brussels sprouts and mushrooms with lettuce salad and avocado

DAY THREE

Breakfast - Omelet with shrimp, sautéed spinach, tarragon and three eggs

Snack - A handful of nuts (no peanuts or cashews)

Lunch - Grilled turkey burger with lettuce, sliced tomatoes, and sautéed mushrooms. Kale chips on the side.

Snack - Sliced peppers with hummus (not made from chickpeas or beans)

Dinner - Baked cod over Bok Choy and mixed greens

Drinks allowed over the three days

One cup of unsweetened black coffee per day

Unsweetened green and/or herbal tea in
unlimited amounts

A minimum of 64 ounces of water a day (about
8 cups)

Chapter 6

Sample Meal Plan for a 7-Day Sugar Detox

The 7-day sugar detox is based on the "Good Foods" and "Foods to Avoid" list in Chapter 4. You can use any combination of foods from the "Good Foods" list in building your plate. Make sure to build your plate in this order:

Proteins

Fats

Vegetables

Make sure that you are eating small meals regularly throughout the day. Arrange your eating similar to the 3 day sugar detox:

Breakfast

Snack

Lunch

Snack

Dinner

Also, make sure to follow the "Good Foods" list diligently in order to get the most out of your 7-day sugar detox.

The next chapter contains special bonus tips to help you maximize your sugar detox results.

Chapter 7

Seven Day Sugar Detox Bonus Tips

Drink more fluids

Try your best to drink three liters of water every day. Be creative by drinking herbal teas, spring water, water with lime, vegetable juice along with straight purified water.

Lemon juice to start your day

Drink one 8 ounce glass of warm or room temperature lemon juice in the morning to activate the digestive process and cleanse your system.

Here's how you make this lemon juice drink:

Ingredients

8 ounces warm or room temperature purified water

1/2 lemon – make sure it's an organic lemon

Directions

Squeeze half a lemon into the 8 ounce glass of water and drink.

Note: Using an organic lemon and purified water is recommended because you are using this drink to flush toxins from your body. The cleaner the food and drink the better the results.

Eat every two to three hours

In order to maintain good blood sugar levels eat every two or three hours.

Exercise regularly

Working out for at least an hour a day is great for your overall health. It aids your sugar detox by raising your heart rate and improving the circulation of blood in your body which in turn creates sweat which releases toxins from the body.

Be mindful when eating

Try to chew your food 14 times before swallowing. When you bring mindfulness to the inner process of digestion you create harmony inside and out.

To learn more about Mindfulness I would recommend checking out Yesenia Chavan's *Mindfulness for Beginners* book on Amazon.

Raw foods

Rather than cooked food try going with raw food. Raw food contains more enzymes and nutrients that assist your body in functioning at an optimum level.

Meditation

You might be wondering what meditation has to do with a sugar detox. Think of it this way. The mind has a powerful ability to affect our overall well-being. As an example, someone that wants to lose weight but suffers from depression can inhibit their own weight loss goals just by the way they think, even if they are working out vigorously every day.

It is important to keep your mind peaceful and clean during your sugar detox. This assists your body in releasing the damaging effects of sugar and embracing a new way of eating. Start your day with a 30 minute meditation session every day.

To learn more about Meditation I would also recommend Yesenia Chavan's *Meditation for Beginners* book also available on Amazon.

Chapter 8

Symptoms and Benefits of a Sugar Detox

So, a sugar detox seems easy enough don't you think? It should be a 'piece of cake' right? Not! Professionals agree that your cravings will disagree with you on how easy this diet is.

Will it be uncomfortable at first? Yes.

Will it be easy? No.

Studies show that kicking the sugar habit can be harder than quitting cocaine. The fact that sugar is so easily accessible makes it even worse.

Symptoms

During a sugar detox you will likely experience the following symptoms for the first day or two:

Headaches

Flu like symptoms

Lethargy

Difficulty sleeping

Diarrhea/Constipation

Skin breakouts

Rashes

Gas, bloating

Body odor

Bad breath

More irritable than normal

Overly sensitive

The importance of a "healing crisis"

Nutritionists, physiotherapists and others involved in health related fields will tell you that feeling worse can actually mean you're getting better. The non-desirable symptoms you might experience on a detox are called a "healing crisis" and usually only last the first few days of a detox.

Remember, our bodies clean themselves from the inside out. This might mean some pretty intense scrubbing and disinfecting. That is why it is perfectly natural to take a few steps back before moving forward.

Benefits

Your cravings for sugar will increase, peaking at around 3-4 days. It will take all of your willpower not to dive head first into a bucket of sherbet or stuff your face with strawberries coated in granulated goodness. So why do it?

When the Sugar Detox Diet is over you will have:

Lost fat

Rejuvenated your skin with the years you thought you lost

Cleared up acne that you've been fighting since the addiction started

Decreased your eczema

Increased your sense of taste so that healthy foods start tasting better. You will also find that you crave healthier foods more often

Reduced your sugar cravings so that sugary treats start losing their appeal

Increased your energy so you feel consistently energetic

Regular bowel movements

Less depression

Better sleep

An increased sense of wellbeing

A feeling of pride for having created a healthy foundation for your life where you are no longer a slave to sugar

By introducing quality proteins into your diet alongside healthy fats and carbs via the Sugar Detox Diet it will not only change the way your palate reacts to food, it will change your habits around your meals as well.

Chapter 9

The Difference Between Natural and Artificial Sweeteners

What is a natural sweetener?

A natural sweetener is one that has not been altered much from its natural state and that actually comes from nature.

The only kind of sugar that is beneficial for us is all-natural sugar found in living fruits, vegetables, trees, herbs, nuts, seeds and roots. Why? Because this is all our body was designed for.

Humans have consumed these natural sugars for numerous decades. The body knows how to work with them and has no problem breaking them down into useable energy.

Honey, molasses, maple syrup, and green leaf stevia are examples of natural sweeteners that have been consumed for hundreds of years.

What is a naturally derived sweetener?

"Naturally derived" means that an ingredient in the sweetener originated in nature. It is unclear however how far back in the processing the ingredient was a whole, natural item. Naturally derived ingredients no longer resemble their natural form.

The word "natural" is not regulated in many markets. We instinctively think that "natural" means healthy but normally the "natural" ingredient has been manipulated so much from its natural form that it no longer contains the health benefits that we would assume it has.

What is an artificial sweetener?

An artificial sweetener is a man-made, chemically engineered compound that is normally used as a low-calorie sweetener that replaces sugar. It is a highly refined modern factory made sweetener that is scientifically proven to be worse for you than sugar and fructose.

Since artificial sweeteners are quite modern, man-made and haven't been around for numerous decades, the body has a hard time appropriately digesting them.

Artificial sweeteners can be found in many foods and beverages marked "sugar-free," "diet," "low-fat," or "non-fat." Sodas, candy, chewing gum, ice cream, yogurt and fruit juices are a few examples of foods and beverages that contain added or artificial sweeteners.

It is important to realize that artificial sweeteners can be misleading. For example, in the world of weight loss, an artificial sweetener can appear to be a good thing because it adds virtually zero calories to your diet. Plus, you only need a tiny amount to add a punch of sweetness to your food or favorite beverage.

High fructose corn syrup is a man-made sweetener made by the food industry that spikes blood sugar levels virtually higher than any other carbohydrate. It is often considered the worst carb ever carrying with it a long list of negative health consequences.

Natural sweeteners

Use these natural sweeteners in very limited quantities AFTER the 21 day, 7 day or 3 day sugar detox:

Brown sugar

Cane juice

Cane juice crystals

Cane sugar

Coconut nectar

Coconut sugar/crystals

Date sugar

Date syrup

Dates

Fruit juice

Fruit juice concentrate

Honey

Maple syrup

Molasses

Palm sugar

Raw sugar

Stevia (green leaf or extract)

Turbinado sugar

Naturally derived sweeteners

Please remember that naturally derived sweeteners can contain good and bad qualities. For example Xylitol has beneficial properties for your teeth whereas corn syrup can be damaging to the body if the corn syrup is infused with HCFS fructose. To stay safe, stick with the natural sweeteners ONLY in limited quantities after your sugar detox.

Agave

Agave nectar

Barley malt

Beet sugar

Brown rice

Syrup

Buttered syrup

Caramel

Carob syrup

Corn syrup

Corn syrup solids

Demerara sugar

Dextran

Dextrose

Diastatic malt

Diastase

Ethyl maltol

Fructose

Glucose

Glucose solids

Golden sugar

Golden syrup

Grape sugar

Invert sugar

Lactose

Levulose

Light brown sugar

Maltitol

Malt syrup

Maltodextrin

Maltose

Mannitol

Muscovado

Refiner's syrup

Sorbitol

Sorghum syrup

Sucrose

Tagatose

Treacle

Yellow sugar

Xylitol

...other sugar alcohols that normally end in "-ose"

Artificial sweeteners

It is best to AVOID these artificial sweeteners ENTIRELY:

High-fructose corn syrup

Acesulfame

K/Acesulfame Potassium

Aspartame

Saccharine

Stevia, white/bleached

Sucralose

Chapter 10

Monitoring Your Sugar

Listen to your body. You might find it trying to warn you when your blood sugar level may be getting dangerously out of balance. How will your body let you know?

You may get intense cravings for sweets, sugar or even breads and pastas when your levels are too low. This is the surest sign that your body is telling you that it wants sugar to lift its spirits

You might get very tired after eating or even light-headed if you miss a meal.

You might find yourself drinking more coffee than normal to keep yourself going throughout the day thinking the caffeine will help keep you alert and functioning.

You may find that losing weight is extremely hard for you and you might not really understand why.

You may notice that eating sweets doesn't really hit the spot and relieve the craving you had to fill the appetite of your sweet tooth.

You can take control!

Don't worry, you can get control! There are many things you can do to get control of your wavering blood sugar:

Eat more animal proteins like eggs, fish, and chicken. These convert to glucose after a little work from your liver and they deliver energy all day and not just in sudden bursts like simple sugars do.

Eliminate simple sugars to avoid those insulin spikes and to keep the energy flow consistent.

Eat complex carbohydrates. These are harder for the body to break down than simple sugars are. They, therefore, give energy for longer periods of time.

Eat more fiber

Ingest good fats rich in essential fatty acids

Commit to the sugar detox diet and don't give in when it gets tough!

Chapter 11

Dining Out During the Detox

Who says a sugar free lifestyle means you can't eat out? Go 'all American' at your favorite burger joint! Feel free to enjoy that big beef patty, just hold the bun and get it wrapped in lettuce. For salads, eat them with a little lemon, vinegar, and oil.

Going for Italian? Avoid pasta, breaded meats, and bread in general. Don't worry, there is more good food left to choose from! Help yourself to grilled chicken, shrimp and veggies or healthy salads as well.

With Indian food skip the rice and naan and double-check the spice rubs to make sure there is no flour in them. Watch out for Tandoori meats too, as they are often times marinated in yogurt.

With Japanese, worry most about the rice: white or brown. Nothing fried and none of the imitation crab sticks. Remember too that many of the sauces in Japanese food contain sugar. Stick with sashimi and broiled fish. Both are okay as long as you don't add soy sauce.

Mexican food is a great option! You can't do the tortilla chips, beans or rice but you can do the meats, salsa and guacamole!

With Thai try to stay away from anything with noodles or that is 'peanut' flavored. Curry however is your friend! Coconut milk based dishes are okay too as long as you skip the rice.

Unfortunately, Chinese is a 'no go'. Many of the sauces have hidden sugars cooked in. MSG is also regularly used in the dishes. Unless you know the chefs in the restaurants really well, avoid Chinese during your detox.

Chapter 12

Reintroducing Sugar

You've officially gotten through 'the cleanse' and you are now sugar free. So, what do you do now? Of course you don't want to ruin all of your hard work by running to your local bakery and stuffing your face full of donuts. You feel great; better than you have in years. So, how do you reintroduce sugar back into your life without letting it take over?

Start by understanding the difference between natural and artificial sweeteners. Make sure to use only natural sweeteners when reintroducing sugar into your diet again. Choose natural sweeteners like brown sugar, honey, and maple syrup. Remember to use them sparingly. After all, pure granulated sugar is 99% sugar, brown sugar is 97% sugar and even honey is 82% sugar. What's the best alternative? If you can stand it, molasses is the best choice.

Add one sweet thing at a time. Choose one food and eat it at every meal for 24 hours along with all of your normal detox foods and keep track of how you feel. The idea is to reintroduce only one potentially problematic food at a time.

Then remove that food for the next two days and see how you feel. Make note of any of the following changes for the next 72 hours: energy, mood, headaches, mental clarity, appetite, bloating, gas or diarrhea.

The notes you keep will help you know whether you have sensitivity to the food you just reintroduced. Don't add anything else to your diet until you know how that particular sugary food works in your system.

It is not recommended to reintroduce gluten-filled grains like wheat, barley and rye. Also, avoid reintroducing pasteurized dairy and unfermented soy products.

Add foods back into your diet bit by bit. Eat starchy foods only on days that you've been most active. This will help you break those sugars down effectively so they will put the least amount of strain on your body.

Keep avoiding foods bought in packages and refined foods like pastas, breads, cereals as well as products made with flour. All of these are sugary foods that will cause more problems for you later. They contain 'hidden' sugars disguised as something else. Don't be fooled by the '100% whole grain label. That doesn't necessarily mean that it's sugar free.

Say 'no' to candy and choose a healthier option instead. This includes chewing gum since most gum is over 50% sugar!

Dried fruits are tricky. You'd think they are okay because they are fruit right? Wrong. They are like compact sugar bombs waiting to go off inside you if you eat too many. Not only will they help dehydrate you, they will cause insulin spikes in your body as well. You can eat them in extremely limited amounts but don't consume more than that.

Sodas are the enemy. One 355 ml (12 ounce) can of your favorite soda will force your body to deal with 42 grams of added sugar. That is the equivalent of 10.5 teaspoons of sugar in just one can of pop!

It goes without saying that cakes and cookies should be avoided as well, simply because granulated sugar is one of the main baking ingredients. Watch out for jams and spreads also as most of them have a high sugar content. Even peanut butter is 10% sugar.

Salad dressings can be a source of hidden sugars as well. Shoot for a simple mix of lemon, lime, extra virgin olive oil and a dash of vinegar instead of your normal salad dressing. Chances are the prepackaged stuff is higher in sugar content than you thought.

Avoid alcohol. It's sugar in disguise. If you have a drink, do it with food to give your body everything it needs to break down the sugar in a healthy way.

The best substitutes to try during your sugar cravings

The bad news is, if you give in and use 'sugar' to quiet the nagging sugar beast inside of you, it will only get worse. The desire for sugar will only get bigger and stronger by eating sugar. It's a vicious cycle.

So what do you do when you have to do something to calm the beast?

Try dark chocolate. If eaten a few times a week dark chocolate will help prevent hardening of your arteries. It will also improve blood flow and lower blood pressure. With the increased blood flow that it causes it can lower your risk of stroke and improve cognitive thinking.

Chocolate contains phenylethylamine (PEA), a chemical that your body releases when you fall in love so it can actually make you *feel* better. Chocolate even has a little bit of caffeine for a 'pick me up' if you are feeling sluggish.

It's full of antioxidants which help protect against cancer and it's also full of theobromine, a bitter alkaloid of the cacao plant which has been proven to help harden tooth enamel. Its glycemic index is low which means your body won't react with huge insulin spikes to try to accommodate the chocolate.

Though they aren't sweet, try sunflower seeds or pistachios. Not only are they packed full of nutrients, the act of cracking them open and eating each seed or nut one at a time can be a stress reliever and can help distract the sugar monster from taking over.

After the detox is over eat fresh fruits instead of sugary substitutes. Avoid bananas, mangos, and pineapples as they are high in sugar but citrus fruits and berries are a great alternative. In fact, an 'apple a day' can 'help keep the sugar beast at bay.'

Have a cup of green tea. Its bitter taste can help shatter the craving. Plus, it's an anti-inflammatory so it can help your body and mind deal with the stress response. The more you use it to help calm your craving the better it will work.

Give fructooligosaccharides a try. Though they are simple sugars they have a minimal effect on blood sugar levels and can even help good bacteria in the intestines. You'll find this type of sugar in onions, garlic, jicama, chicory root, leeks and even asparagus. The Jerusalem artichoke and the Blue Agave plant contain the highest concentrations of fructooligosaccharides.

Exercise is a great stress buster. When you start getting overwhelmed with the desire to stuff your face with cakes and pies put on your runners and get moving. A long jog or just a quick work out at the gym can do wonders to silence the sugar cravings.

Chapter 13

How to Maintain a Limited Sugar Lifestyle

When you've made the change to live your life as 'sugar-free' as possible you'll start noticing sugar everywhere; the cookies that come with your sandwich, the icing on the cake, the packets of sugar that come with your coffee etc.

Western society encourages the sugar addiction. Sugar is added to our foods without us even knowing it. It is pushed into our lives with the age old saying, "A little won't hurt anything....right?"

Well... remember that a little WILL hurt you. A little sugar WILL help feed the addiction you just broke away from.

This is a commitment you've made with yourself. Remind yourself of that every day. You aren't depriving yourself of something good; you are saving your body from something that is highly addictive and dangerous to your health.

Tips for sticking with your limited sugar lifestyle

Enjoy your food. Just because you've made a decision not to have that giant piece of cake doesn't mean that you can't enjoy the food you are eating. Make your meals well rounded and satisfying. Don't forget to savor every bite. The conscious decision to enjoy what you are eating even if it isn't loaded with sugar will make a huge difference in how you experience food.

Toss the bad stuff. Get rid of everything in your home that could potentially feed the addiction and fill your house with healthy foods that encourage you to stay on track.

Plan ahead. Bring your meals with you when you go out and have healthy snacks ready and waiting.

Add healthy rituals to your lifestyle. How about a walk after dinner? Make it that special thing that you do for yourself. Don't make it dependent on someone else.

Take care of yourself. Block out time to reflect on your needs and desires and how you are feeling. Celebrate yourself. Manage your stress as best as you can. Don't let it get unmanageable. Find something that helps you relax like yoga, meditation or going for a run in order to keep your stress under control.

Read food labels. Just because the marketing tactics on the front say the food is healthy doesn't mean that it is. Understand how to read labels. Study up on what each category on a food label means and how it relates to your diet. Be a smart shopper and make sure you aren't bringing anything into your home that shouldn't be there.

Don't cook twice. If you have a family and you are the only one making the commitment to a limited sugar lifestyle, do yourself a favor and don't tempt yourself with cooking something that you know you shouldn't have. Your family doesn't have to make the same choices as you, but you don't have to cook something you know is bad for them either. Be creative by making healthy food fun and delicious!

The recipes in the next chapter will help you with this!

Chapter 14

Sugar Free 'Detox Friendly" 30 MINUTE Recipes

These recipes are taken from my Sugar Free Recipes book on Amazon

BREAKFAST RECIPES

Eggs Nested in Shiitake Mushrooms and Sautéed Chard

Shiitake mushrooms give a nice earthy flavor to this nutritious breakfast!

Ingredients

2 tablespoons extra virgin olive oil

½ cup onion, chopped

½ pound fresh chard, sliced (separate the chard ribs from the leaves)

3 large shiitake mushrooms sliced into 1/4-inch slices

2 medium or large eggs

Salt and pepper to taste

Directions

Add olive oil to a medium saucepan and heat.

Add the onions, chard ribs and mushrooms. Sauté on medium heat for five minutes or until the onions turn opaque.

Add the chard leaves to the saucepan. Toss with tongs or use a spatula to ensure all the ingredients are mixed together well. When thoroughly mixed, spread over the bottom of the pan evenly.

Add one or two eggs to the center of the pan. This creates the nest. Reduce heat to medium low and cook the eggs 3-4 minutes. When the egg whites are cooked through they are finished. Remove from heat and transfer to serving plate.

Bacon Wrapped Omelet Mini's

These tasty little omelet bites are packed with protein and flavor. They make a perfectly nutritious breakfast!

Ingredients

2 cups chicken, diced and cooked

12 thin bacon slices

4 eggs, large

12 egg whites, large

2 cups chopped spinach

½ medium green pepper, finely chopped

½ medium red pepper, finely chopped

Seasoning salt to taste

Directions

Preheat the oven to 350°F

Cook the bacon in a pan over medium high heat until it is cooked through. Make sure it doesn't get crispy. Roughly five minutes.

Spray a muffin tin with non-stick cooking spray then wrap one piece of bacon around the outer edges of each tin.

In a medium sized bowl, scramble the four large eggs with the twelve egg whites. Add the red and green peppers, diced chicken, spinach and seasoning salt. Combine.

Pour the mixture into each muffin tin lined with bacon. Use a spoon or ladle to transfer the mixture.

Bake until the eggs are fluffy and slightly brown on top about 25 minutes.

You can top this dish with avocado or change things up by adding different ingredients like mushrooms, onions or sausage.

LUNCH RECIPES

Dijon Broccoli Chicken

This is a very flavorful dish that includes broccoli and chicken drenched in a delicious tangy sauce.

Ingredients

1 pound chicken breasts cut into thin strips

½ cup chicken broth

6 teaspoons Dijon mustard

1 tablespoon extra virgin olive oil

4 cups broccoli florets

2 cloves garlic, minced

Salt and pepper to taste

Directions

Heat the olive oil in a large skillet on medium heat. Add the garlic, and broccoli. Cook the broccoli until it is crisp on the outside yet tender on the inside. Remove the broccoli from the skillet and cover.

Add the chicken to the skillet and cook until it is crispy and cooked through.

Add the chicken broth to the chicken.

Bring to a boil then reduce the heat to medium low.

Add the mustard and stir well to mix.

Return the broccoli to the skillet and stir to mix. Cook until heated through. Serve warm.

Low-Carb Turkey and Egg Lettuce Wraps

This is an excellent low-carb snack that's extra tasty!

Ingredients

8 lettuce leaves. Romaine lettuce

8 slices of deli-style turkey meat

8 large eggs, boiled

Directions

In a medium pot, add all eight eggs and cover with water.

Turn the heat to high and boil the eggs for 5-10 minutes.

Remove pot from heat and run cold water over the hard-boiled eggs.

Peel the eggs.

Take eight lettuce leaves and wash them under cold running water.

Place a lettuce leaf on a serving plate and add a slice of deli style turkey meat on top of it. Cut a hard-boiled egg into slices and place it on top of the turkey.

Roll the lettuce leaf with the turkey and the egg to form a wrap. Serve.

DINNER RECIPES

Balsamic Lemon Garlic Salmon

Salmon is an excellent source of omega-3's. The blend of balsamic vinegar, lemon and garlic go perfectly with the salmon.

Ingredients

8 ounces sockeye salmon fillets

2 tablespoons balsamic vinegar

2 tablespoons olive oil

1 tablespoon fresh lemon juice from one lemon

1 garlic clove minced

Salt to taste

Directions

Preheat the broiler.

In a medium dish, add salt, balsamic vinegar, lemon juice, garlic, and the olive oil. Whisk the ingredients together.

Dip the fish into the mixture and place on a baking sheet.

Brush additional moisture onto the fish.

Make sure the oven rack is 4 inches from the heat source.

Place the fish in the oven and broil 4 to 6 minutes turning midway.

Fish should flake when finished. Serve sprinkled with balsamic vinegar.

Shiitake Mushrooms and Chicken Lettuce Wraps

Shiitake mushrooms have been used as a medicine in China for more than 6000 years. They are full of health promoting properties.

Ingredients

1 pound ground chicken

1 teaspoon cornstarch

1 teaspoon extra virgin olive oil

2 green onions chopped

4 ounces sliced shiitake mushrooms

2 teaspoons seasoned rice vinegar

½ teaspoon toasted sesame oil

1 yellow bell pepper diced

3 celery sticks diced

1 head Bib lettuce rinsed, leaves separated

Salt and pepper to taste

Directions

In a large bowl, add the ground chicken and corn starch. Stir to mix and set aside to marinate.

Heat a wok or large skillet to medium heat. When the wok or skillet is hot, add the olive oil.

Add the green onions and the shiitake mushrooms and cook them for a minute or two.

Increase the heat to high and add the ground chicken and cornstarch. Stir and break up the chicken to make sure it cooks evenly all the way through, 5-7 minutes.

Add seasoned rice vinegar, sesame oil and diced bell pepper and celery.

Remove from heat. Adjust seasonings to taste.

Create cups with the lettuce and scoop the chicken mixture into the lettuce. Serve warm.

Options: Add a few chili pepper flakes to the oil as it is heating. Top with some fresh cilantro leaves. Experiment with other meats.

SALAD RECIPES

Kale with Tomatoes and Garlic

Garlic contains antioxidants that can boost your immune system and improve your skin. It also supports the respiratory and circulatory system and prevents inflammation due to the anti-inflammatory properties that it contains.

Ingredients

Kale.....1 pound, hard stems removed, chopped coarsely

Extra-virgin olive oil.....2 teaspoons

Garlic cloves.....4 thinly sliced

Vegetables stock or chicken broth.....1/2 cup

Cherry tomatoes.....1 cup halved

Lemon.....1 tablespoon lemon juice

Black pepper.....1/8 teaspoon

Directions

In a large pan on medium heat, add olive oil and garlic. Sauté until garlic is lightly toasted (about 1 or 2 minutes).

Add the Kale, vegetable stock or chicken broth, and cover to simmer.

Lower the heat to medium low and cook until kale wilts (about five minutes).

Remove the lid, add the tomatoes, and cook until kale is tender.

Transfer the kale to a medium bowl and add lemon juice and salt and pepper to taste. Serve immediately.

Bacon and Broccoli Salad

Broccoli is loaded with vitamin K and vitamin C! Just one serving of broccoli gives you your daily requirement of these two vitamins.

Serves 2

Ingredients

2 rashers bacon, chopped into matchstick slices (Rashers bacon is thinly sliced ham that is broiled or fried)

1 head broccoli, chopped

1 avocado

½ cup sliced almonds

2 tablespoons Dijon mustard

2 tablespoons sherry vinegar

2 tablespoons olive oil

Directions

In a small skillet on medium high heat, add the matchstick chopped rashers bacon. (Note: rashers bacon is thinly sliced ham that is broiled or fried)

Let the bacon get crisp and browned. Rashers should warm through. You may need a teaspoon of oil in the pan especially if the rasher is precooked and you are reheating.

In a small bowl, add the mustard, vinegar, and olive oil. Whisk together.

Chop the broccoli and put it into a medium bowl.

Pour the dressing over the broccoli and stir.

Toast the almonds and add to the broccoli salad.

Mix the ingredients together and top with the crispy bacon rashers. Serve immediately.

Tuna Nicoise Salad

Tuna Nicoise salad typically incorporates potatoes but those have been excluded in order to adhere to the sugar detox diet.

Serves 2

Ingredients

325 grams fresh tuna loin

100 grams green beans, chopped

3 eggs, hard boiled

3 Baby Gem lettuces –Baby Gem is a mini version of Romaine lettuce

200 grams cherry tomatoes

2 tablespoons balsamic vinegar

A handful of fresh basil leaves, chopped

Juice of half a lemon

6 tablespoons olive oil, divided

Dressing:

50 grams black olives

5 marinated anchovy fillets

1 tablespoon balsamic vinegar

1 garlic clove

4 tablespoons extra virgin olive oil

Juice of half a lemon

Salt to taste

Directions

Dressing:

Put the olives, anchovies and garlic into a bowl and mash them to get a rough paste. Add the olive oil, lemon juice and balsamic vinegar. Set aside.

Salad:

Cook the greens beans in lightly salted water until tender. About 5 minutes. Drain. Pour cold water over them then set aside.

Bring a small pot of water to a boil and add the eggs. Cook for 10 minutes to make hard boil. Drain. Pour cold water over the eggs then peel them and set them aside.

In a frying pan heat 2 tablespoons of oil then add the tomatoes and cook for about 1 minute. Drizzle with 1 tablespoon of balsamic vinegar.

Season with salt to taste. Stir. Remove from heat and top with basil.

For the tuna, heat a non-stick frying pan on high then turn down to medium and add 1 tablespoon of olive oil. Season the tuna with salt on both sides. Allow it to sear for 4 minutes until the underside is brown. Turn it over and sear on the other side for 4 minutes until brown. Cooking the tuna for 4 minutes on each side will give you very rare tuna. If you want your tuna a little less rare then cook it for 2 minutes more per side. If you want your tuna well done add 4 more minutes to each side. When the tuna is done, set it aside to rest for a few minutes.

To serve, mix the remaining balsamic vinegar with the remaining oil and lemon juice. Add the Baby Gem lettuce to the bowl and mix together.

Place 1 spoonful of dressing into 2 serving bowls. Put the tomato mix on top of the dressing then add some green beans to each bowl. Cut the tuna in half and place on top of the beans.

Wedge the Baby Gem lettuce around the sides of the bowl. Cut the eggs in half and put them between the tuna and lettuce.

Pour the remaining dressing over each serving. Enjoy!

SIDE DISH RECIPES

Roasted Zucchini with Garlic

An easy, tasty dish!

Ingredients

1 pound zucchini, each cut lengthwise twice, and then cut in half across the middle

1 tablespoon fresh minced garlic clove

¼ cup olive oil

1 teaspoon Herbes de Provence

Salt and freshly ground black pepper to taste

Directions

Preheat the oven to 450 degrees and place the rack on the top.

Place the zucchini on a baking sheet skin down.

In a small bowl, mix the garlic and olive oil together then brush the garlic oil over the zucchini.

Bake the zucchini on the top rack for five minutes and check to see if it is browning on the top. If not continue to bake a couple more minutes. Continue to check for a nice golden brown.

Once you see the golden brown appear, you can remove from the oven and put into a bowl. Add the Herbes de Provence then salt and pepper to taste. Serve immediately.

Bok Choy with Almonds

Bok Choy has the highest concentration of beta-carotene and vitamin A than any other cabbage? It also makes a great side dish for your other dinner favorites.

Ingredients

2 tablespoons olive oil

1 cup green onions, finely chopped

3 garlic cloves, finely chopped

1 pound baby Bok Choy, rinsed, larger leaves separated from base

1/2 teaspoon dark sesame oil

1/2 cup sliced almonds, chopped and roasted

Salt to taste

Directions

In a large frying pan or wok on medium high heat, add the extra virgin olive oil.

Sauté the onions and garlic and let them cook for about one minute then add the bok choy.

Sprinkle the ingredients with the sesame oil and salt. Cover with a tight fitting lid.

The Bok Choy should cook down in about 3 minutes. It will wilt and resemble spinach.

Remove the cover, lower the heat to simmer and stir.

Allow the Bok Choy to cook a couple more minutes and transfer to a serving bowl.

Add the roasted almonds stir and serve warm.

SOUP RECIPES

Egg Drop Chicken Soup

Try this low carbohydrate soup for lunch. It will leave you feeling satisfied and you will not need to snack between meals.

Ingredients

1 large egg

¼ teaspoon white pepper

2 cups chicken stock

1 tablespoon chopped chives

Directions

In a bowl, whisk the egg then set aside. Boil the chicken broth and briskly stir in the whisked egg leaving long tendrils in the soup.

Season with chives and white pepper.

Optional: Feel free to add one carrot, one celery stick and 1 yellow onion to your broth if you like.

Cauliflower Soup

An excellent soup for a cold winter's day!

Ingredients

2 stalks celery, chopped

1 onion, chopped

¾ cup shredded carrots

2 tablespoons olive oil

1 head cauliflower, coarsely chopped

6 cups chicken broth

Ground black pepper to taste

Directions

In a large saucepan on medium heat, add the olive oil and allow it to heat to a warm temperature. Sauté the celery, carrots, and onions until the onions turn opaque. Remove from heat and set aside.

In a colander, steam the cauliflower until tender. Remove and strain then mash the cauliflower and add to the large saucepan of celery, carrots, and onions. Return the pan to the stove and cook on medium heat.

Add the chicken broth and stir ingredients together. Pepper to taste and simmer for another 15 minutes. Serve immediately.

SNACK RECIPES

Pesto Dip with Walnuts and Cilantro

This dip can be served with vegetables, on fish or chicken and as a sandwich spread.

Ingredients

3 cups cilantro

2 ½ ounces light sour cream

1/3 cup toasted walnuts, chopped

1 garlic clove

½ ounce juice from fresh lemon

¼ cup olive oil

½ teaspoon salt

Directions

In a food processor, add the cilantro, walnuts, and garlic. Chop the ingredients for 30 seconds. Add the olive oil in a steady stream while the processor is still running.

Add the sour cream, salt, and lemon juice. Pulse the processor to combine all the ingredients together.

Serve immediately or refrigerate to cool.

Note: You can freeze this mixture for up to one month or you can refrigerate it for up to five days.

Bacon Wrapped Sea Scallops

Yummy!

Ingredients

1 teaspoon cracked black pepper

2 tablespoons olive oil

1 lemon – the juice of one lemon

1 thick slice packed 12/pound smoked bacon

1 pound sea scallops

Directions

In a small bowl, add the olive oil, pepper and lemon. Whisk the ingredients together and pour over the scallops in a shallow dish. Cover with plastic wrap and put in the fridge to marinate for at least an hour.

Preheat the broiler.

When scallops have marinated remove from the fridge and wrap each scallop with a slice of thick bacon, about 1/2 inch strips.

Insert a toothpick to pinch the bacon onto the scallop or use a skewer and place at least three scallops on a skewer.

Place on the broiler pan, broil until golden brown and flip over to brown other side. Make sure the bacon cooks to desired crispness then remove from broiler and serve immediately.

Cut each piece of bacon diagonally into thirds then wrap one piece of bacon around each stuffed jalapeno. Poke the toothpick through the bacon and jalapeno to secure. Place on the cookie sheet.

Bake 20 minutes or until the bacon is crispy and jalapenos are soft. Serve warm.

Conclusion

Congratulations on finishing the book!

I pour my heart into every book and make every effort to help you achieve your diet and health goals.

I hope this book has given you all the information you need to apply the sugar detox to your life TODAY!

May this detox be the start of a fantastic, energetic and healthy new life for you!

Other books by Gina Crawford

Sugar Free Recipes

Paleo for Beginners

Mediterranean Diet for Beginners

Mediterranean Diet Cookbook

DASH Diet for Beginners

DASH Diet Recipes

5:2 Diet for Beginners

5:2 Diet Recipes

Available on Amazon

About Gina Crawford

Understanding what it takes to live a healthy lifestyle, eat right, achieve your goal weight and love your life shouldn't be complicated. Your time is valuable and the last thing you need is to tackle a 300 page book on how to get your health, weight and life on track. If you're like most people, you just want the facts in bite-sized, easy to understand pieces that you can apply to your life TODAY!

My name is Gina Crawford. I am a health and "all things natural" enthusiast, author, mother and wife. Years ago I was overweight, exhausted, unhappy and desperately aching for a better life. One day, gruelingly tired of my situation, I started researching everything I could on health and transforming my life. I often felt overwhelmed by the amount of information and the changes I had to make, but I persevered and managed to turn my life around one book and one bite at a time.

Now I'm determined to share what I've learned in an easy, non-overwhelming, "no fluff, no filler, straight to the point" kind of way that will allow others to achieve maximum results in a short amount of time.

I am passionate about every book I write and my goal with each book is to make it simple and concise yet power-packed with the necessary information you need to transform your life. I have learned first-hand the incredible value of healing ourselves with natural organic foods, natural remedies, exercise and a positive mindset.

When I'm not writing, I love spending time with my family, cooking, walking, biking and reading.

My hope is that my books will help you live a healthier, better, more passionate, alive life!

Happy reading!

Made in the USA
Lexington, KY
23 March 2017